My Diabetic Recipe Book

*A Full Set of Easy & Delicious Diabetic-Friendly
Recipes for Beginners*

Valerie Blanchard

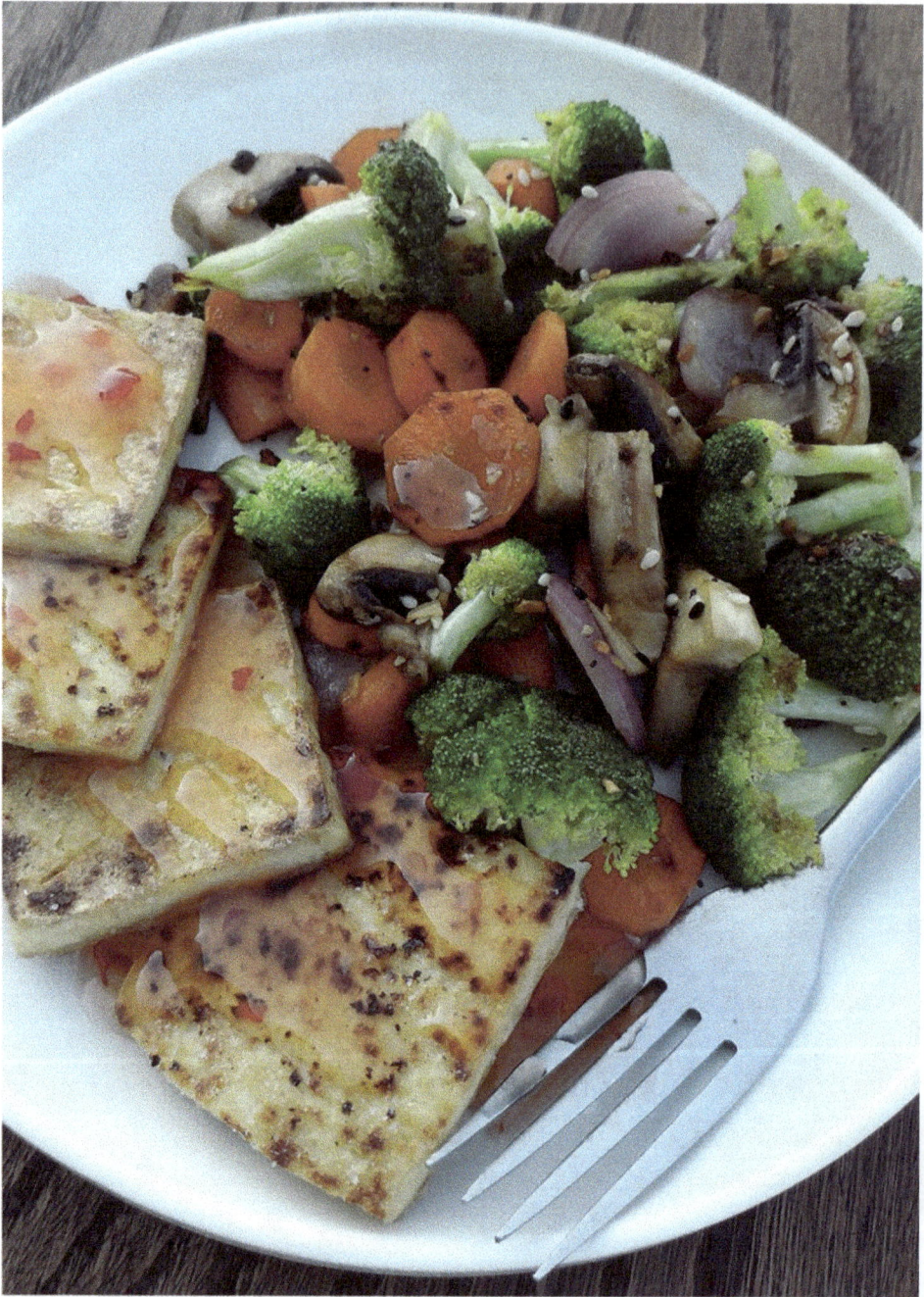

Table of Contents

Blueberry Buns

Preparation Time: 10 minutes

Cooking Time: 12 minutes

Servings: 6

Ingredients:

- 240g all-purpose flour
- 50g granulated sugar
- 8g baking powder
- 2g of salt
- 85g chopped cold butter
- 85g of fresh blueberries
- 3g grated fresh ginger
- 113 ml whipping cream
- 2 large eggs
- 4 ml vanilla extract
- 5 ml of water

Directions:

1. Put sugar, flour, baking powder and salt in a large bowl.

2. Put the butter with the flour using a blender or your hands until the mixture resembles thick crumbs.

3. Mix the blueberries and ginger in the flour mixture and set aside

4. Mix the whipping cream, 1 egg and the vanilla extract in a different container.

5. Put the cream mixture with the flour mixture until combined.

6. Shape the dough until it reaches a thickness of approximately 38 mm and cut it into eighths.

7. Spread the buns with a combination of egg and water. Set aside Preheat the air fryer set it to 180C.

8. Place baking paper in the preheated inner basket and place the buns on top of the paper. Cook for 12 minutes at 180C, until golden brown

Nutrition: Calories: 105; Fat: 1.64g; Carbohydrates: 20.09g; Protein: 2.43g; Sugar: 2.1g; Cholesterol: 0mg

Cauliflower Potato Mash

Preparation Time: 30 minutes Servings: 4

Cooking Time: 5 minutes

Ingredients:

- 2 cups potatoes, peeled and cubed
- 2 tbsp. butter
- ¼ cup milk
- 10 oz. cauliflower florets
- ¾ tsp. salt

Directions:

1. Add water to the saucepan and bring to boil.
2. Reduce heat and simmer for 10 minutes.
3. Drain vegetables well. Transfer vegetables, butter, milk, and salt in a blender and blend until smooth.
4. Serve and enjoy.

Nutrition: Calories 128; Fat 6.2 g; Sugar 3.3 g; Protein 3.2 g; Cholesterol 17 mg

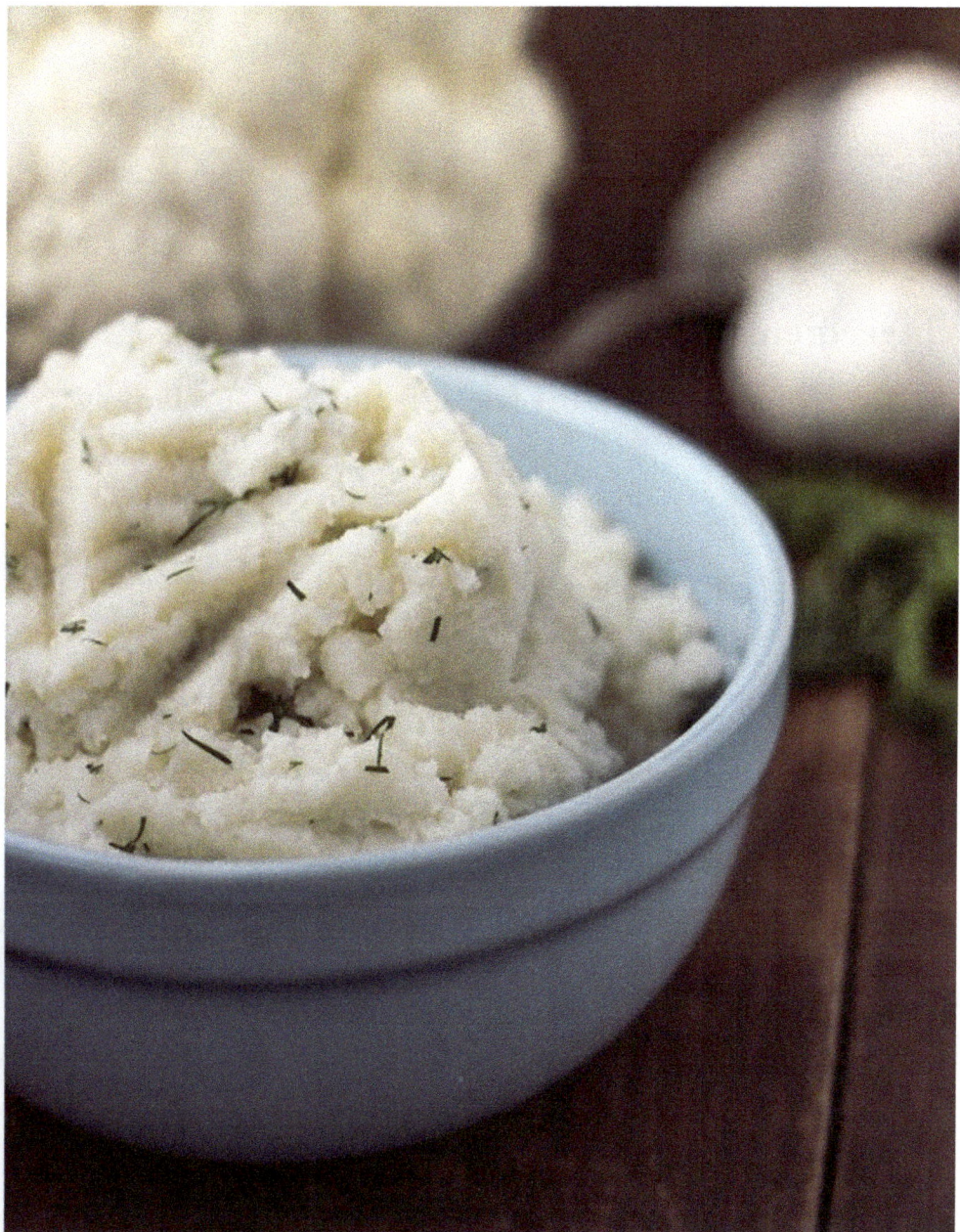

French toast in Sticks

Preparation Time: 5 minutes

Cooking Time: 10 minutes

Servings: *4*

Ingredients:

- 4 slices of white bread, 38 mm thick, preferably hard
- 2 eggs
- 60 ml of milk
- 15 ml maple sauce
- 2 ml vanilla extract
- Nonstick Spray Oil
- 38g of sugar
- 3ground cinnamon
- Maple syrup, to serve
- Sugar to sprinkle

Directions:

1. Cut each slice of bread into thirds making 12 pieces. Place sideways

2. Beat the eggs, milk, maple syrup and vanilla.

3. Preheat the air fryer, set it to 175C.

4. Dip the sliced bread in the egg mixture and place it in the preheated air fryer. Sprinkle French toast generously with oil spray.

5. Cook French toast for 10 minutes at 175C. Turn the toast halfway through cooking.

6. Mix the sugar and cinnamon in a bowl.

7. Cover the French toast with the sugar and cinnamon mixture when you have finished cooking.

8. Serve with Maple syrup and sprinkle with powdered sugar

Nutrition: Calories 128; Fat 6.2 g; Carbohydrates 16.3 g; Sugar 3.3 g; Protein 3.2 g; Cholesterol 17 mg

Muffins Sandwich

Preparation Time: 2 minutes

Cooking Time: 10 minutes

Servings: *1*

Ingredients:

- Nonstick Spray Oil
- 1 slice of white cheddar cheese
- 1 slice of Canadian bacon
- 1 English muffin, divided
- 15 ml hot water
- 1 large egg
- Salt and pepper to taste

Directions:

1. Spray the inside of an 85g mold with oil spray and place it in the air fryer.

2. Preheat the air fryer, set it to 160C.

3. Add the Canadian cheese and bacon in the preheated air fryer.

4. Pour the hot water and the egg into the hot pan and season with salt and pepper.

5. Select Bread, set to 10 minutes.

6. Take out the English muffins after 7 minutes, leaving the egg for the full time.

7. Build your sandwich by placing the cooked egg on top of the English muffing and serve

Nutrition: Calories 400; Fat 26g; Carbohydrates 26g; Sugar 15 g; Protein 3 g; Cholesterol 155 mg

Bacon BBQ

Preparation Time: 2 minutes

Cooking Time: 8 minutes

Servings: _2_

Ingredients :

- 13g dark brown sugar
- 5g chili powder
- 1g ground cumin
- 1g cayenne pepper
- 4 slices of bacon, cut in half

Directions:

1. Mix seasonings until well combined.
2. Dip the bacon in the dressing until it is completely covered. Leave aside.
3. Preheat the air fryer, set it to 160C.
4. Place the bacon in the preheated air fryer
5. Select Bacon and press Start/Pause.

Nutrition: Calories: 1124; Fat: 72g; Carbohydrates: 59g; Protein: 49g; Sugar: 11g; Cholesterol: 77mg

Stuffed French toast

Preparation Time: 4 minutes

Cooking Time: 10 minutes

Servings: *1*

Ingredients:

- 1 slice of brioche bread,
- 64 mm thick, preferably rancid
- 113g cream cheese
- 2 eggs
- 15 ml of milk
- 30 ml whipping cream
- 38g of sugar
- 3g cinnamon
- 2 ml vanilla extract
- Nonstick Spray Oil
- Pistachios chopped to cover
- Maple syrup, to serve

Directions:

1. Preheat the air fryer, set it to 175C.

2. Cut a slit in the middle of the muffin.

3. Fill the inside of the slit with cream cheese. Leave aside.

4. Mix the eggs, milk, whipping cream, sugar, cinnamon, and vanilla extract.

5. Moisten the stuffed French toast in the egg mixture for 10 seconds on each side.

6. Sprinkle each side of French toast with oil spray.

7. Place the French toast in the preheated air fryer and cook for 10 minutes at 175C

8. Stir the French toast carefully with a spatula when you finish cooking.

9. Serve topped with chopped pistachios and acrid syrup.

Nutrition: Calories: 159; Fat: 7.5g; Carbohydrates: 25.2g; Protein: 14g; Sugar: 0g; Cholesterol: 90mg

Chili Chicken Wings

Preparation Time: 10 minutes

Cooking Time: 1 hour 10 minutes

Servings: *4*

Ingredients:

- 2 lbs. chicken wings
- 1/8 tsp. paprika
- 1/2 cup coconut flour
- 1/4 tsp. garlic powder
- 1/4 tsp. chili powder

Directions:

1. Preheat the oven to 400 F/ 200 C.
2. In a mixing bowl, add all **Ingredients** except chicken wings and mix well.
3. Add chicken wings to the bowl mixture and coat well and place on a baking tray.
4. Bake in preheated oven for 55-60 minutes.
5. Serve and enjoy.

Nutrition: Calories 440; Fat 17.1 g; Carbohydrates 1.3 g; Sugar 0.2 g; Protein 65.9 g; Cholesterol 202 mg

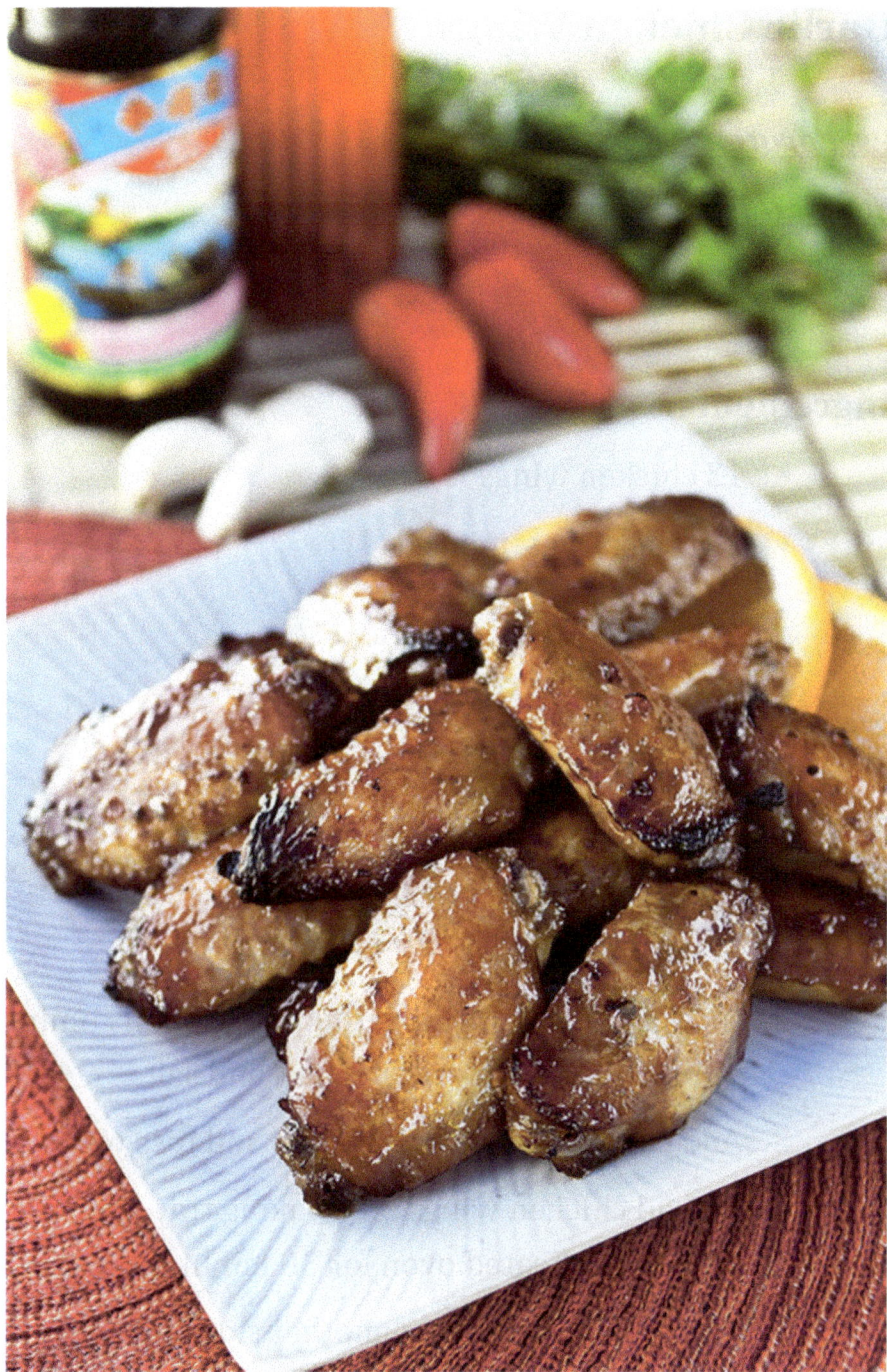

Garlic Chicken Wings

Preparation Time: 10 minutes

Cooking Time: 55 minutes

Servings: *6*

Ingredients:

- 12 chicken wings
- 2 garlic cloves, minced
- 3 tbsp. ghee
- 1/2 tsp. turmeric
- 2 tsp. cumin seeds

Directions:

1. Preheat the oven to 425 F/ 215 C.
2. In a large bowl, mix together 1 teaspoon cumin, 1 tbsp. ghee, turmeric, pepper, and salt.
3. Add chicken wings to the bowl and toss well.
4. Spread chicken wings on a baking tray and bake in preheated oven for 30 minutes.
5. Turn chicken wings to another side and bake for 8 minutes more.

6. Meanwhile, heat remaining ghee in a pan over medium heat.

7. Add garlic and cumin to the pan and cook for a minute.

8. Remove pan from heat and set aside.

9. Remove chicken wings from oven and drizzle with ghee mixture

10. Bake chicken wings 5 minutes more.

11. Serve and enjoy.

Nutrition: Calories 378; Fat 27.9 g; Carbohydrates 11.4 g; Sugar 0 g; Protein 19.7 g; Cholesterol 94 mg

Spinach Cheese Pie

Preparation Time: 10 minutes

Cooking Time: 40 minutes

Servings: _8_

Ingredients:

- 6 eggs, lightly beaten
- 2 boxes frozen spinach, chopped
- 2 cup cheddar cheese, shredded
- 15 oz. cottage cheese
- 1 tsp. salt

Directions:

1. Preheat the oven to 375 F/ 190 C.
2. Spray an 8*8-inch baking dish with cooking spray and set aside.
3. In a mixing bowl, combine together spinach, eggs, cheddar cheese, cottage cheese, pepper, and salt.
4. Pour spinach mixture into the prepared baking dish and bake in preheated oven for 10 minutes.

5. Serve and enjoy.

__Nutrition:__ Calories 229; Fat 14 g; Carbohydrates 5.4 g; Sugar 0.9 g; Protein 21 g; Cholesterol 157 mg

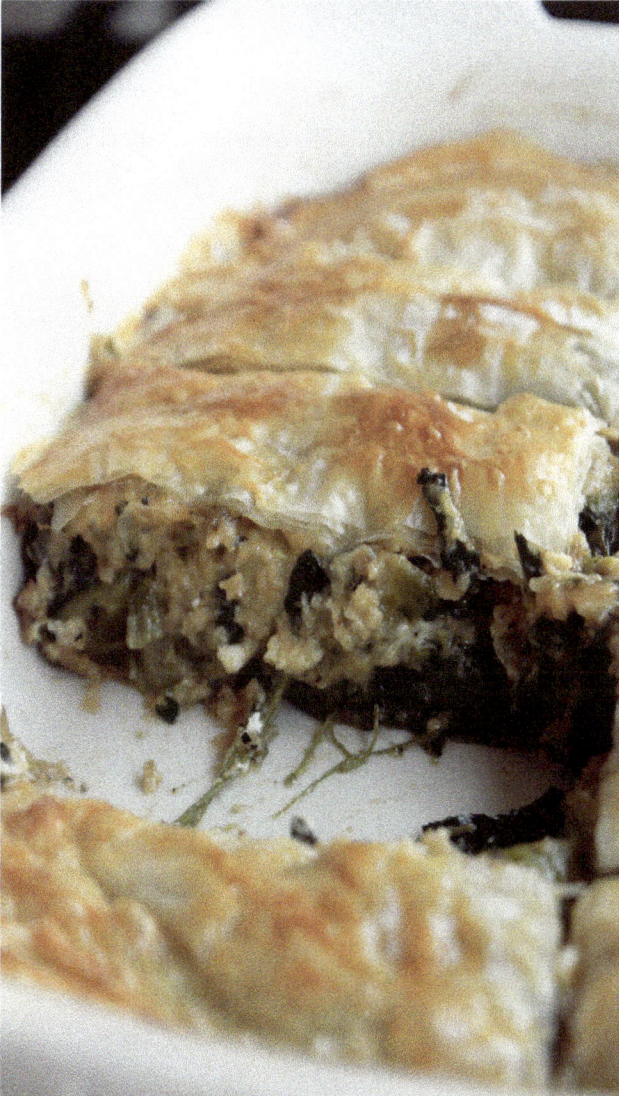

Tasty Harissa Chicken

Preparation Time: 10 minutes

Cooking Time: 4 hours 10 minutes

Servings: *4*

Ingredients:

- 1 lb. chicken breasts, skinless and boneless
- 1/2 tsp. ground cumin
- 1 cup harissa sauce
- 1/4 tsp. garlic powder
- 1/2 tsp. kosher salt

Directions:

1. Season chicken with garlic powder, cumin, and salt.
2. Place chicken to the slow cooker.
3. Pour harissa sauce over the chicken.
4. Cover slow cooker with lid and cook on low for 4 hours.
5. Remove chicken from slow cooker and shred using a fork.

6. Return shredded chicken to the slow cooker and stir well.

7. Serve and enjoy.

Nutrition: Calories 232; Fat 9.7 g; Carbohydrates 1.3 g; Sugar 0.1 g; Protein 32.9 g; Cholesterol 101 mg

Roasted Balsamic Mushrooms

Preparation Time: 10 minutes

Cooking Time: 50 minutes

Servings: *4*

Ingredients:

- 8 oz. mushrooms, sliced
- 1/2 tsp. thyme
- 2 tbsp. balsamic vinegar
- 2 tbsp. extra virgin olive oil
- 2 onions, sliced

Directions:

1. Preheat the oven to 375 F/ 190 C.
2. Line baking tray with aluminum foil and spray with cooking spray and set aside.
3. In a mixing bowl, add all **Ingredients** and mix well.
4. Spread mushroom mixture onto a prepared baking tray.
5. Roast in preheated oven for 45 minutes.
6. Season with pepper and salt.

7. Serve and enjoy.

Nutrition: Calories 96; Fat 7.2 g; Carbohydrates 7.2 g; Sugar 3.3 g; Protein 2.4 g; Cholesterol 0 mg

Roasted Cumin Carrots

Preparation Time: 10 minutes

Cooking Time: 45 minutes

Servings: *4*

Ingredients:

- 8 carrots, peeled and cut into 1/2-inch-thick slices
- 1 tsp. cumin seeds
- 1 tbsp. olive oil
- 1/2 tsp. kosher salt

Directions:

1. Preheat the oven to 400 F/ 200 C.
2. Line baking tray with parchment paper.
3. Add carrots, cumin seeds, olive oil, and salt in a large bowl and toss well to coat.
4. Spread carrots on a prepared baking tray and roast in preheated oven for 20 minutes.
5. Turn carrots to another side and roast for 20 minutes more.
6. Serve and enjoy.

Nutrition: Calories 82; Fat 3.6 g; Carbohydrates 12.2 g; Sugar 6 g; Protein 1.1 g; Cholesterol 0 mg

Tasty & Tender Brussels Sprouts

Preparation Time: 10 minutes

Cooking Time: 35 minutes

Servings: _4_

Ingredients:

- 1 lb. Brussels sprouts, trimmed cut in half
- ¼ cup balsamic vinegar
- 1 onion, sliced
- 1 tbsp. olive oil

Directions:

1. Add water in a saucepan and bring to boil.
2. Add Brussels sprouts and cook over medium heat for 20 minutes. Drain well.
3. Heat oil in a pan over medium heat.
4. Add onion and cook until softened. Add sprouts and vinegar and stir well and cook for 1-2 minutes.
5. Serve and enjoy.

Nutrition: Calories 93; Fat 3.9 g; Carbohydrates 13 g; Sugar 3.7 g; Protein 4.2 g; Cholesterol 0 mg

Sautéed Veggies

__Preparation Time:__ 10 minutes

__Cooking Time__: 15 minutes

Servings: *4*

Ingredients*:*

- 1/2 cup mushrooms, sliced
- 1 zucchini, diced
- 1 squash, diced
- 2 1/2 tsp. southwest seasoning
- 3 tbsp. olive oil

Directions:

1. In a medium bowl, whisk together southwest seasoning, pepper, olive oil, and salt.
2. Add vegetables to a bowl and mix well to coat.
3. Heat pan over medium-high heat.
4. Add vegetables in the pan and sauté for 5-7 minutes.
5. Serve and enjoy.

Nutrition: Calories 107; Fat 10.7 g; Carbohydrates 3.6 g; Sugar 1.5 g; Protein 1.2 g; Cholesterol 0 mg

Mustard Green Beans

Preparation Time: 10 minutes

Cooking Time: 20 minutes

Servings: *4*

Ingredients:

- 1 lb. green beans, washed and trimmed
- 1 tsp. whole grain mustard
- 1 tbsp. olive oil
- 2 tbsp. apple cider vinegar
- 1/4 cup onion, chopped

Directions:

1. Steam green beans in the microwave until tender.
2. Meanwhile, in a pan heat olive oil over medium heat.
3. Add the onion in a pan sauté until softened.
4. Add water, apple cider vinegar, and mustard in the pan and stir well.
5. Add green beans and stir to coat and heat through.

6. Season green beans with pepper and salt.

7. Serve and enjoy.

Nutrition: Calories 71; Fat 3.7 g; Carbohydrates 8.9 g; Sugar 1.9 g; Protein 2.1 g; Cholesterol 0 mg

Zucchini Fries

Preparation Time: 10 minutes

Cooking Time: 40 minutes

Servings: *4*

Ingredients:

- 1 egg
- 2 medium zucchinis, cut into fry's shape
- 1 tsp. Italian herbs
- 1 tsp. garlic powder
- 1 cup parmesan cheese, grated

Directions:

1. Preheat the oven to 425 F/ 218 C.
2. Spray a baking tray with cooking spray and set aside.
3. In a small bowl, add egg and lightly whisk it.
4. In a separate bowl, mix together spices and parmesan cheese.
5. Dip zucchini fries in egg then coat with parmesan cheese mixture and place on a baking tray.

6. Bake in preheated oven for 25-30 minutes. Turn halfway through.

7. Serve and enjoy.

Nutrition: Calories 184; Fat 10.3 g; Carbohydrates 3.9 g; Sugar 2 g; Protein 14.7 g; Cholesterol 71 mg

Broccoli Nuggets

Preparation Time: 10 minutes

Cooking Time: 25 minutes

Servings: *4*

Ingredients:

- 2 cups broccoli florets
- 1/4 cup almond flour
- 2 egg whites
- 1 cup cheddar cheese, shredded
- 1/8 tsp. salt

Directions:

1. Preheat the oven to 350 F/ 180 C.
2. Spray a baking tray with cooking spray and set aside.
3. Using potato masher breaks the broccoli florets into small pieces.
4. Add remaining **Ingredients** to the broccoli and mix well.
5. Drop 20 scoops onto baking tray and press lightly into a nugget shape.

6. Bake in preheated oven for 20 minutes.

7. Serve and enjoy.

Nutrition: Calories 148; Fat 10.4 g; Carbohydrates 3.9 g; Sugar 1.1 g; Protein 10.5; Cholesterol 30 mg

Zucchini Cauliflower Fritters

Preparation Time: 10 minutes

Cooking Time: 15 minutes

Servings: *4*

Ingredients:

- 2 medium zucchinis, grated and squeezed
- 3 cups cauliflower florets
- 1 tbsp. coconut oil
- 1/4 cup coconut flour
- 1/2 tsp. sea salt

Directions:

1. Steam cauliflower florets for 5 minutes.
2. Add cauliflower into the food processor and process until it looks like rice.
3. Add all **Ingredients** except coconut oil to the large bowl and mix until well combined.
4. Make small round patties from the mixture and set aside.
5. Heat coconut oil in a pan over medium heat.

6. Place patties in a pan and cook for 3-4 minutes on each side.

7. Serve and enjoy.

Nutrition: Calories 68 Fat 3.8 g; Carbohydrates 7.8 g; Sugar 3.6 g; Protein 2.8 g; Cholesterol 0 mg

Roasted Chickpeas

Preparation Time: 10 minutes

Cooking Time: 30 minutes

Servings: *4*

Ingredients:

- 15 oz. can chickpeas, drained, rinsed and pat dry
- 1/2 tsp. paprika
- 1 tbsp. olive oil
- 1/2 tsp. pepper
- 1/2 tsp. salt

Directions:

1. Preheat the oven to 450 F/ 232 C.
2. Spray a baking tray with cooking spray and set aside.
3. In a large bowl, toss chickpeas with olive oil, paprika, pepper, and salt.
4. Spread chickpeas on a prepared baking tray and roast in preheated oven for 25 minutes. Stir every 10 minutes.

5. Serve and enjoy.

Nutrition: Calories 158; Fat 4.8 g; Carbohydrates 24.4 g; Sugar 0 g; Protein 5.3 g; Cholesterol 0 mg

Peanut Butter Mousse

Preparation Time: 10 minutes

Cooking Time: 10 minutes

Servings: *2*

Ingredients:

- 1 tbsp. peanut butter
- 1 tsp. vanilla extract
- 1 tsp. stevia
- 1/2 cup heavy cream

Directions:

1. Add all **Ingredients** into the bowl and whisk until soft peak forms.
2. Spoon into the **Serving** bowls and enjoy.

Nutrition: Calories 157; Fat 15.1 g; Carbohydrates 5.2 g; Sugar 3.6 g; Protein 2.6 g; Cholesterol 41 mg

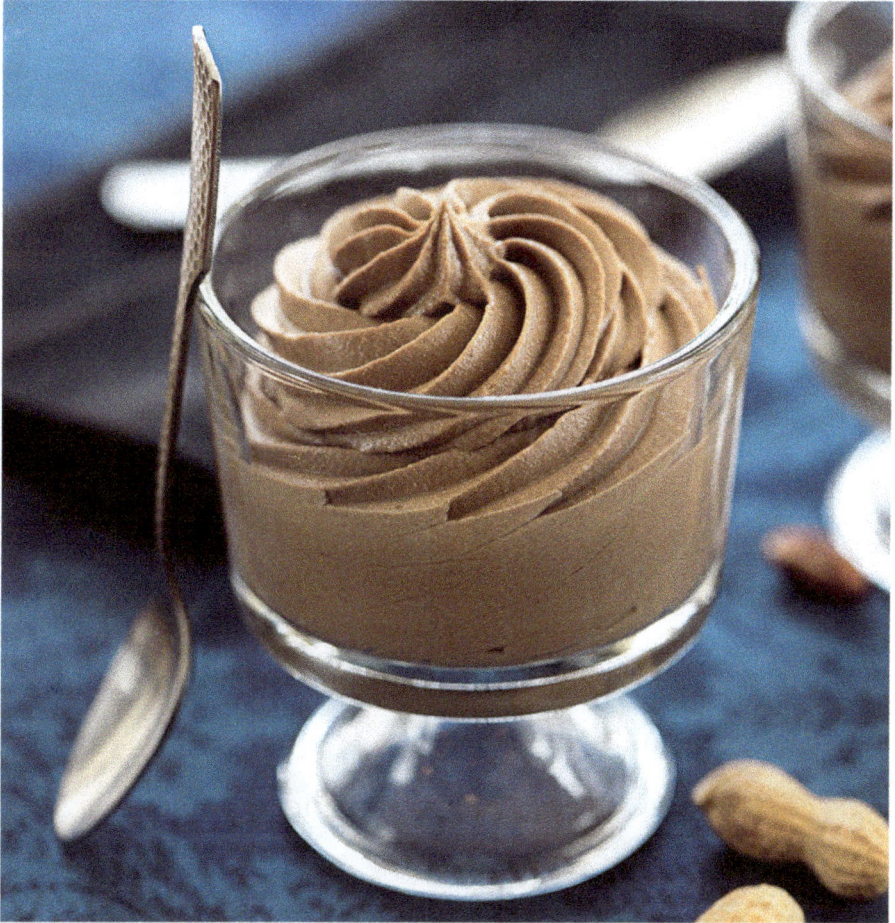

Coffee Mousse

Preparation Time: 10 minutes

Cooking Time: 20 minutes

Servings: *8*

Ingredients:

- 4 tbsp. brewed coffee
- 16 oz. cream cheese, softened
- 1/2 cup unsweetened almond milk
- 1 cup whipping cream
- 2 tsp. liquid stevia

Directions:

1. Add coffee and cream cheese in a blender and blend until smooth.
2. Add stevia, and milk and blend again until smooth.
3. Add cream and blend until thickened.
4. Pour into the **Serving** glasses and place in the refrigerator.
5. Serve chilled and enjoy.

Nutrition: Calories 244; Fat 24.6 g; Carbohydrates 2.1 g; Sugar 0.1 g; Protein 4.7 g; Cholesterol 79 mg

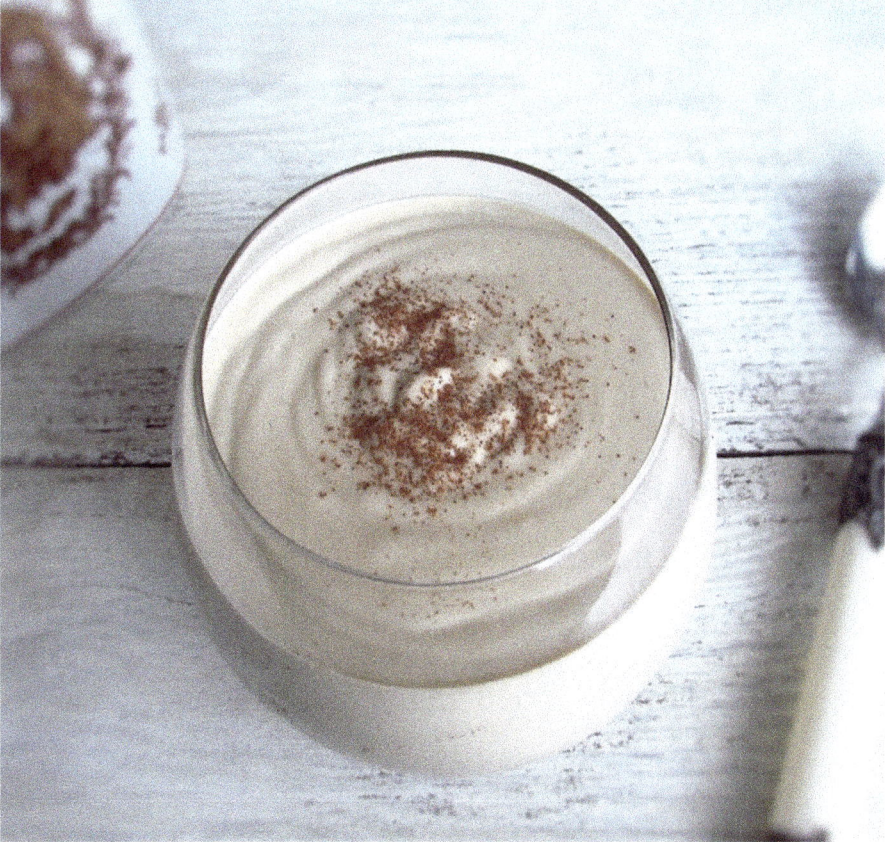

Wild Rice and Black Lentils Bowl

Preparation Time: 10 minutes

Cooking Time: 50 minutes

Servings: *4*

Ingredients:

- Wild rice
- 2 cups wild rice, uncooked
- 4 cups spring water
- ½ teaspoon salt
- 2 bay leaves
- Black lentils
- 2 cups black lentils, cooked
- 1 ¾ cups coconut milk, unsweetened
- 2 cups vegetable stock
- 1 teaspoon dried thyme
- 1 teaspoon dried paprika
- ½ of medium purple onion; peeled, sliced
- 1 tablespoon minced garlic
- 2 teaspoons creole seasoning

- 1 tablespoon coconut oil
- Plantains
- 3 large plantains, chopped into ¼-inch-thick pieces
- 3 tablespoons coconut oil
- Brussels sprouts
- 10 large brussels sprouts, quartered
- 2 tablespoons spring water
- 1 teaspoon sea salt
- ½ teaspoon ground black pepper

Directions:

1. Prepare the rice: take a medium pot, place it over medium-high heat, pour in water, and add bay leaves and salt.

2. Bring the water to a boil, then switch heat to medium, add rice, and then cook for 30–45 minutes or more until tender.

3. When done, discard the bay leaves from rice, drain if any water remains in the pot, remove it from heat, and fluff by using a fork. Set aside until needed.

4. While the rice boils, prepare lentils: take a large pot, place it over medium-high heat and when hot, add onion and cook for 5 minutes or until translucent.

5. Stir garlic into the onion, cook for 2 minutes until fragrant and golden, then add remaining **Ingredients** for the lentils and stir until mixed.

6. Bring the lentils to a boil, then switch heat to medium and simmer the lentils for 20 minutes until tender, covering the pot with a lid.

7. When done, remove the pot from heat and set aside until needed.

8. While rice and lentils simmer, prepare the plantains: chop them into ¼-inch-thick pieces.

9. Take a large skillet pan, place it over medium heat, add coconut oil and when it melts, add half of the plantain pieces and cook for 7–10 minutes per side or more until golden-brown.

10. When done, transfer browned plantains to a plate lined with paper towels and repeat with the remaining plantain pieces; set aside until needed.

11.　Prepare the sprouts: return the skillet pan over medium heat, add more oil if needed, and then add brussels sprouts.

12.　Toss the sprouts until coated with oil, and then let them cook for 3–4 minutes per side until brown.

13.　Drizzle water over sprouts, cover the pan with the lid, and then cook for 3–5 minutes until steamed.

14.　Season the sprouts with salt and black pepper, toss until mixed, and transfer sprouts to a plate.

15.　Assemble the bowl: divide rice evenly among four bowls and then top with lentils, plantain pieces, and sprouts.

16.　Serve immediately.

Nutrition: Calories: 333; Carbohydrates: 49.2 g; Fat: 10.7 g; Protein: 6.2 g

Alkaline Spaghetti Squash Recipe

Preparation Time: 10 minutes

Cooking Time: 30 minutes

Servings: 4

Ingredients:

- 1 spaghetti squash
- Grapeseed oil
- Sea salt
- Cayenne powder (optional)
- Onion powder (optional)

Directions:

1. Preheat your oven to 375°f
2. Carefully chop off the ends of the squash and cut it in half.
3. Scoop out the seeds into a bowl.
4. Coat the squash with oil.
5. Season the squash and flip it over for the other side to get baked. When properly baked, the outside of the squash will be tender.

6. Allow the squash to cool off, then, use a fork to scrape the inside into a bowl.

7. Add seasoning to taste.

8. Dish your alkaline spaghetti squash!

Nutrition: Calories: 672; Carbohydrates: 65 g; Fat: 47 g; Protein: 12 g

Dairy-Free Fruit Tarts

Preparation Time: 15 minutes

Cooking Time: 15 minutes

Servings: *2*

Ingredients:

1 cup Coconut Whipped Cream

½ Easy Shortbread Crust (dairy-free option)

Fresh mint Sprigs

½ cup mixed fresh Berries

Directions:

1. Grease two 4" pans with detachable bottoms. Pour the shortbread mixture into pans and firmly press into the edges and bottom of each pan. Refrigerate for 15 minutes.

2. Loosen the crust carefully to remove from the pan.

3. Distribute the whipped cream between the tarts and evenly spread to the sides. Refrigerate for 1-2 hours to make it firm.

4. Use the berries and sprig of mint to garnish each of the tarts

Nutrition: Fat: 28.9g; Carbs: 8.3g; Protein: 5.8g; Calories: 306

Spaghetti Squash with Peanut Sauce

Preparation Time: 15 minutes

Cooking Time: 15 minutes

Servings: *4*

Ingredients:

- 1 cup cooked shelled edamame; frozen, thawed
- 3-pound spaghetti squash
- ½ cup red bell pepper, sliced
- ¼ cup scallions, sliced
- 1 medium carrot, shredded
- 1 teaspoon minced garlic
- ½ teaspoon crushed red pepper
- 1 tablespoon rice vinegar
- ¼ cup coconut aminos
- 1 tablespoon maple syrup
- ½ cup peanut butter
- ¼ cup unsalted roasted peanuts, chopped
- ¼ cup and 2 tablespoons spring water, divided
- ¼ cup fresh cilantro, chopped

- 4 lime wedges

Directions:

1. Prepare the squash: cut each squash in half lengthwise and then remove seeds.

2. Take a microwave-proof dish, place squash halves in it cut-side-up, drizzle with 2 tablespoons water, and then microwave at high heat setting for 10–15 minutes until tender.

3. Let squash cool for 15 minutes until able to handle. Use a fork to scrape its flesh lengthwise to make noodles, and then let noodles cool for 10 minutes.

4. While squash microwaves, prepare the sauce: take a medium bowl, add butter in it along with red pepper and garlic, pour in vinegar, coconut aminos, maple syrup, and water, and then whisk until smooth.

5. When the squash noodles have cooled, distribute them evenly among four bowls, top with scallions, carrots, bell pepper, and edamame beans, and then drizzle with prepared sauce.

6. Sprinkle cilantro and peanuts and serve each bowl with a lime wedge.

Nutrition: Calories: 419; Carbohydrates: 32.8 g; Fat: 24 g; Protein: 17.6 g

Cauliflower Alfredo Pasta

Preparation Time: 10 minutes

Cooking Time: 30 minutes

Servings: *4*

Ingredients:

- Alfredo sauce
- 4 cups cauliflower florets, fresh
- 1 tablespoon minced garlic
- ¼ cup **Nutrition**al yeast
- ½ teaspoon garlic powder
- ¾ teaspoon sea salt
- ½ teaspoon onion powder
- ½ teaspoon ground black pepper
- ½ tablespoon olive oil
- 1 tablespoon lemon juice, and more as needed for serving
- ½ cup almond milk, unsweetened
- Pasta
- 1 tablespoon minced parsley

- 1 lemon, juiced
- ½ teaspoon sea salt
- ¼ teaspoon ground black pepper
- 12 ounces spelt pasta; cooked, warmed

Directions:

1. Take a large pot half full with water, place it over medium-high heat, and then bring it to a boil.

2. Add cauliflower florets, cook for 10–15 minutes until tender, drain them well, and then return florets to the pot.

3. Take a medium skillet pan, place it over low heat, add oil and when hot, add garlic and cook for 4–5 minutes until fragrant and golden-brown.

4. Spoon garlic into a food processor, add remaining **Ingredients** for the sauce in it, along with cauliflower florets, and then pulse for 2–3 minutes until smooth.

5. Tip the sauce into the pot, stir it well, place it over medium-low heat, and then cook for 5 minutes until hot.

6. Add pasta into the pot, toss well until coated, taste to adjust seasoning, and then cook for 2 minutes until pasta gets hot.

7. Divide pasta and sauce among four plates, season with salt and black pepper, drizzle with lemon juice, and then top with minced parsley.

8. Serve straight away.

Nutrition: Calories: 360; Carbohydrates: 59 g; Fat: 9 g; Protein: 13 g

Sloppy Joe

Preparation Time: 8 minutes

Cooking Time: 12 minutes

Servings: *4*

Ingredients:

- 2 cups kamut or spelt wheat, cooked
- ½ cup white onion, diced
- 1 roma tomato, diced
- 1 cup chickpeas, cooked
- ½ cup green bell peppers, diced
- 1 teaspoon sea salt
- 1/8 teaspoon cayenne pepper
- 1 teaspoon onion powder
- 1 tablespoon grapeseed oil
- 1 ½ cups barbecue sauce, alkaline

Directions:

1. Plug in a high-power food processor, add chickpeas and spelt, cover with the lid, and then pulse for 15 seconds.

2. Take a large skillet pan, place it over medium-high heat, add oil and when hot, add onion and bell pepper, season with salt, cayenne pepper, and onion powder, and then stir until well combined.

3. Cook the vegetables for 3–5 minutes until tender. Add tomatoes, add the pulsed mixture, pour in barbecue sauce, and then stir until well mixed.

4. Simmer for 5 minutes, then remove the pan from heat and serve sloppy joe with alkaline flatbread.

Nutrition: Calories: 333; Carbohydrates: 65 g; Fat: 5 g; Protein: 14 g

Amaretti

Preparation Time: 15 minutes

Cooking Time: 22 minutes

Servings: *2*

Ingredients:

- ½ cup of granulated Erythritol-based Sweetener
- 165g (2 cups) sliced Almonds
- ¼ cup of powdered of Erythritol-based sweetener
- 4 large egg whites
- Pinch of salt
- ½ tsp. almond extract

Directions:

1. Heat the oven to 300° F and use parchment paper to line 2 baking sheets. Grease the parchment slightly.
2. Process the powdered sweetener, granulated sweetener, and sliced almonds in a food processor until it appears like coarse crumbs.

3. Beat the egg whites plus the salt and almond extracts using an electric mixer in a large bowl until they hold soft peaks. Fold in the almond mixture so that it becomes well combined.

4. Drop spoonful of the dough onto the prepared baking sheet and allow for a space of 1 inch between them. Press a sliced almond into the top of each cookie.

5. Bake in the oven for 22 minutes until the sides becomes brown. They will appear jellylike when they are taken out from the oven but will begin to be firms as it cools down.

Nutrition: Fat: 8.8g; Carbs: 4.1g; Protein: 5.3g; Calories: 117

Green Fruit Juice

Preparation Time: 10 minutes

Cooking Time: 0 minutes

Servings: *2*

Ingredients:

- 3 large kiwis, peeled and chopped

- 3 large green apples, cored and sliced

- 2 cups seedless green grapes

- 2 teaspoons fresh lime juice

Directions:

1. Add all **Ingredients** into a juicer and extract the juice according to the manufacturer's method.

2. Pour into 2 glasses and serve immediately.

Nutrition: Calories 304; Total Fat 2.2 g; Saturated Fat 0 g; Protein 6.2 g

Kale Chickpea Mash

Preparation Time: 15 minutes

Cooking Time: 12 minutes

Servings: 1

Ingredients:

- 1 shallot
- 3 tbsp garlic
- A bunch of kale
- 1/2 cup boiled chickpea
- 2 tbsp coconut oil
- Sea salt

Directions:

1. Add some garlic in olive oil
2. Chop shallot and fry it with oil in a nonstick skillet.
3. Cook until the shallot turns golden brown.
4. Add kale and garlic in the skillet and stir well.
5. Add chickpeas and cook for 6 minutes. Add the rest of the **Ingredients** and give a good stir.

6. Serve and enjoy

Nutrition: Calories: 149; Total fat: 8 g; Saturated fat: 1 g; Net Carbohydrates: 13 g; Protein: 4 g; Sugars 6g; Fiber 3g; Sodium 226mg; Potassium 205mg

Quinoa and Apple

The combination of quinoa and apple yields a delicious and filling lunch dish that can be carried to work in your lunch box.

**Preparation Time:** 15 minutes

**Cooking Time**: 12 minutes

Servings: 1

**Ingredients:**

- 1/2 cup quinoa
- 1 apple
- 1/2 lemon
- Cinnamon to taste

**Directions:**

1. Cook quinoa according to the packet **Directions** .
2. Grate the apple and add to the cooked quinoa. Cook for 30 seconds.
3. Serve in a bowl then sprinkle lime and cinnamon. Enjoy.

Nutrition: Calories 229; Total fat: 3.2 g; Net Carbs: 32.3 g; Protein: 6.1 g; Sugars: 4.2 g; Fiber: 3.3 g; Sodium: 35.5 mg; Potassium: 211.8 mg

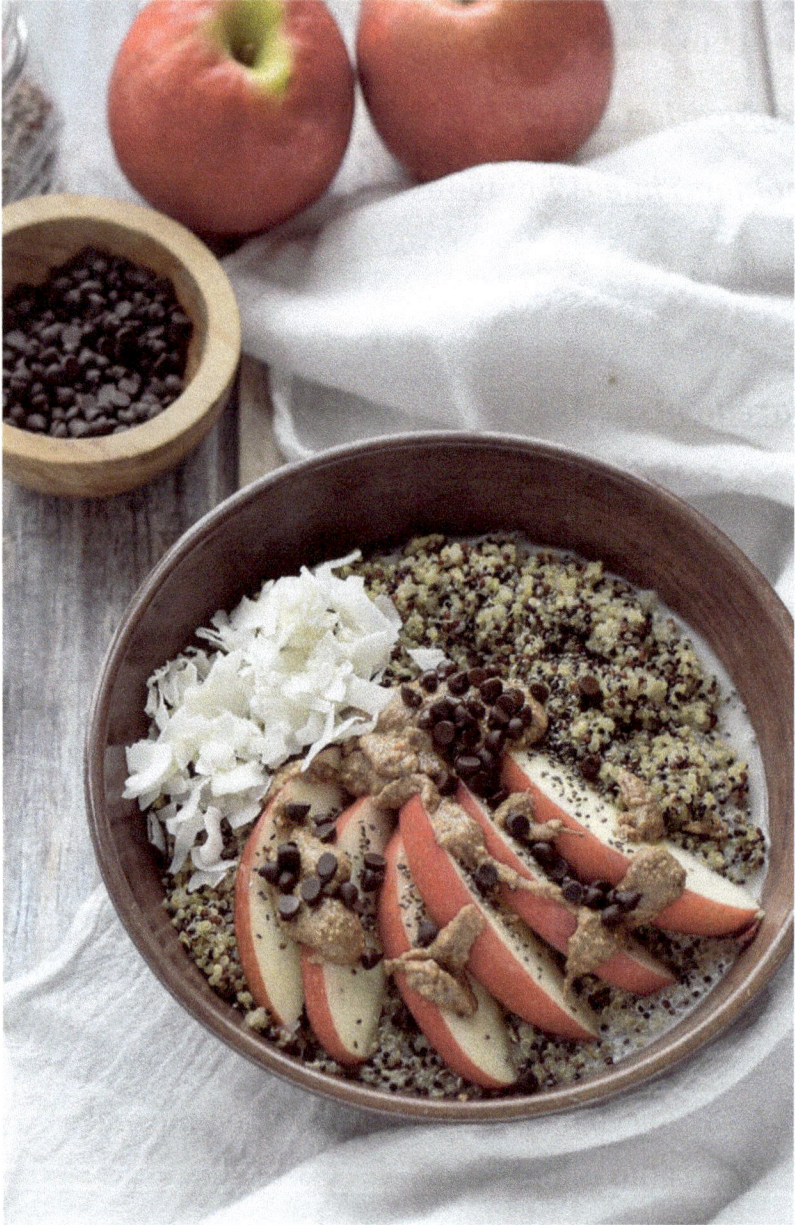

Warm Avo And Quinoa Salad

This is an amazing alkaline quinoa dish that will blow your mind away. It's an easy dish that will be ready in less than 20 minutes.

__Preparation Time:__ 5 minutes

__Cooking Time__: 12 minutes

__Servings:__ 4

__Ingredients:__

- 4 ripe avocados, quartered
- 1 cup quinoa
- 0.9 lb. Chickpeas, drained
- 1 oz flat leaf parsley

__Directions:__

1. Add quinoa in a pot with 2 cups of water. Bring to boil then simmer for 12 minutes or until all the water has evaporated. The grains should be glassy and swollen.

2. Toss the quinoa with all other **Ingredients** and season with salt and pepper to taste.

3. Serve with olive oil and lemon wedges. Enjoy.

Nutrition: Calories: 354; Total fat: 16 g; Saturated fat: 2 g; Net Carbs: 31 g; Protein: 15 g; Sugars: 6 g; Fiber: 15 g; Sodium: 226 mg; Potassium: 205 mg

Tuna Salad

Preparation Time: 15 minutes

Cooking Time: 30 minutes

Servings: 2

Ingredients:

- 2 (5-ounce) cans water packed tuna, drained
- 2 tablespoons fat-free plain Greek yogurt
- Salt and ground black pepper, as required
- 2 medium carrots, peeled and shredded
- 2 apples, cored and chopped
- 2 cups fresh spinach, torn

Directions:

1. In a large bowl, add the tuna, yogurt, salt and black pepper and gently, stir to combine.
2. Add the carrots and apples and stir to combine.
3. Serve immediately.

Nutrition: Calories 306; Total Fat 1.8g; Saturated Fat 0 g; Cholesterol 63 mg; Total Carbs 38 g; Sugar 26 g; Fiber 7.6 g; Sodium 324 mg; Potassium 602 mg; Protein 35.8 g

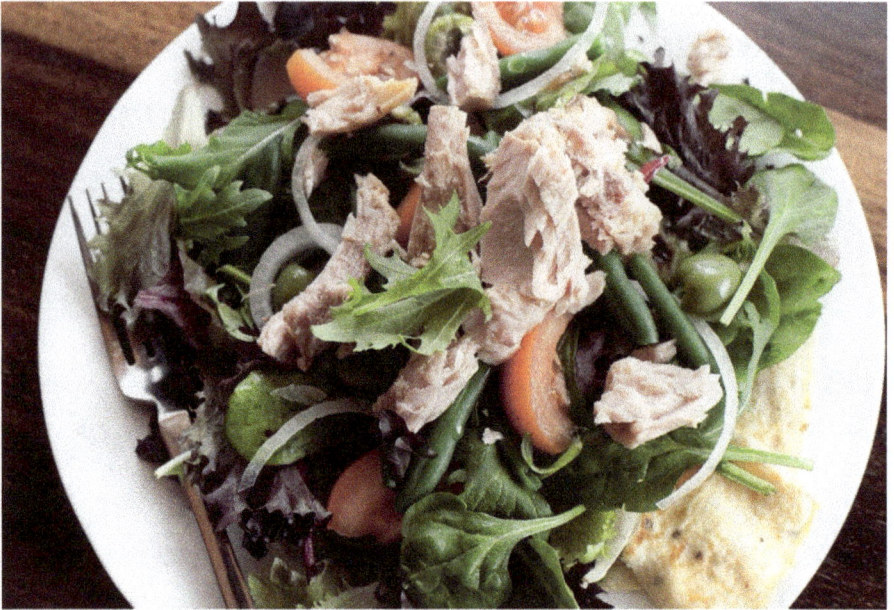

Herring & Veggies Soup

__Preparation Time:__ 15 minutes

__Cooking Time__: 25 minutes

__Servings:__ 5

Ingredients:

- 2 tablespoons olive oil
- 1 shallot, chopped
- 2 small garlic cloves, minced
- 1 jalapeño pepper, chopped
- 1 head cabbage, chopped
- 1 small red bell pepper, seeded and chopped finely
- 1 small yellow bell pepper, seeded and chopped finely
- 5 cups low-sodium chicken broth
- 2 (4-ounce) boneless herring fillets, cubed
- ¼ cup fresh cilantro, minced
- 2 tablespoons fresh lemon juice
- Ground black pepper, as required

- 2 scallions, chopped

Directions:

1. In a large soup pan, heat the oil over medium heat and sauté shallot and garlic for 2-3 minutes.
2. Add the cabbage and bell peppers and sauté for about 3-4 minutes.
3. Add the broth and bring to a boil over high heat.
4. Now, reduce the heat to medium-low and simmer for about 10 minutes.
5. Add the herring cubes and cook for about 5-6 minutes.
6. Stir in the cilantro, lemon juice, salt and black pepper and cook for about 1-2 minutes.
7. Serve hot with the topping of scallion.

Nutrition: Calories 215; Total Fat 11.2g; Saturated Fat 2.1 g; Cholesterol 35 mg; Total Carbs 14.7 g; Sugar 7 g; Fiber 4.5 g; Sodium 152 mg; Potassium 574 mg; Protein 15.1 g

Salmon Soup

Preparation Time: 15 minutes

Cooking Time: 20 minutes

Servings: 4

Ingredients:

- 1 tablespoon olive oil
- 1 yellow onion, chopped
- 1 garlic clove, minced
- 4 cups low-sodium chicken broth
- 1-pound boneless salmon, cubed
- 2 tablespoon fresh cilantro, chopped
- Ground black pepper, as required
- 1 tablespoon fresh lime juice

Directions:

1. In a large pan heat the oil over medium heat and sauté the onion for about 5 minutes.
2. Add the garlic and sauté for about 1 minute.

3. Stir in the broth and bring to a boil over high heat.

4. Now, reduce the heat to low and simmer for about 10 minutes.

5. Add the salmon and soy sauce and cook for about 3-4 minutes.

6. Stir in black pepper, lime juice, and cilantro and serve hot.

Nutrition: Calories 208; Total Fat 10.5 g; Saturated Fat 1.5 g; Cholesterol 50 mg; Total Carbs 3.9 g; Sugar 1.2 g; Fiber 0.6 g; Sodium 121 mg; Potassium 331 mg; Protein 24.4 g

Salmon & Shrimp Stew

Preparation Time: 20 minutes

Cooking Time: 21 minutes

Servings: 6

Ingredients:

- 2 tablespoons olive oil
- 1/2 cup onion, chopped finely
- 2 garlic cloves, minced
- 1 Serrano pepper, chopped
- 1 teaspoon smoked paprika
- 4 cups fresh tomatoes, chopped
- 4 cups low-sodium chicken broth
- 1 pound salmon fillets, cubed
- 1 pound shrimp, peeled and deveined
- 2 tablespoons fresh lime juice
- ¼ cup fresh basil, chopped
- ¼ cup fresh parsley, chopped
- Ground black pepper, as required
- 2 scallions, chopped

Directions:

1. In a large soup pan, melt coconut oil over medium-high heat and sauté the onion for about 5-6 minutes.

2. Add the garlic, Serrano pepper and smoked paprika and sauté for about 1 minute.

3. Add the tomatoes and broth and bring to a gentle simmer over medium heat.

4. Simmer for about 5 minutes.

5. Add the salmon and simmer for about 3-4 minutes.

6. Stir in the remaining seafood and cook for about 4-5 minutes.

7. Stir in the lemon juice, basil, parsley, sea salt and black pepper and remove from heat.

8. Serve hot with the garnishing of scallion.

Nutrition: Calories 271; Total Fat 11 g; Saturated Fat 1.8 g; Cholesterol 193 mg; Total Carbs 8.6 g; Sugar 3.8 g; Fiber 2.1 g; Sodium 273 mg; Potassium 763 mg; Protein 34.7 g

Salmon Curry

Preparation Time: 15 minutes

Cooking Time: 30 minutes

Servings: 6

Ingredients:

- 6 (4-ounce) salmon fillets
- 1 teaspoon ground turmeric, divided
- Salt, as required
- 3 tablespoon olive oil, divided
- 1 yellow onion, chopped finely
- 1 teaspoon garlic paste
- 1 teaspoon fresh ginger paste
- 3-4 green chilies, halved
- 1 teaspoon red chili powder
- 1/2 teaspoon ground cumin
- 1/2 teaspoon ground cinnamon
- ¾ cup fat-free plain Greek yogurt, whipped
- ¾ cup filtered water
- 3 tablespoon fresh cilantro, chopped

Directions:

1. Season each salmon fillet with 1/2 teaspoon of the turmeric and salt.

2. In a large skillet, melt 1 tablespoon of the butter over medium heat and cook the salmon fillets for about 2 minutes per side.

3. Transfer the salmon onto a plate.

4. In the same skillet, melt the remaining butter over medium heat and sauté the onion for about 4-5 minutes.

5. Add the garlic paste, ginger paste, green chilies, remaining turmeric and spices and sauté for about 1 minute.

6. Now, reduce the heat to medium-low.

7. Slowly, add the yogurt and water, stirring continuously until smooth.

8. Cover the skillet and simmer for about 10-15 minutes or until desired doneness of the sauce.

9. Carefully, add the salmon fillets and simmer for about 5 minutes.

10. Serve hot with the garnishing of cilantro.

Nutrition: Calories 242; Total Fat 14.3 g; Saturated Fat 2 g; Cholesterol 51 mg; Total Carbs 4.1 g; Sugar 2 g; Fiber 0.8 g; Sodium 98 mg; Potassium 493 mg; Protein 25.4 g

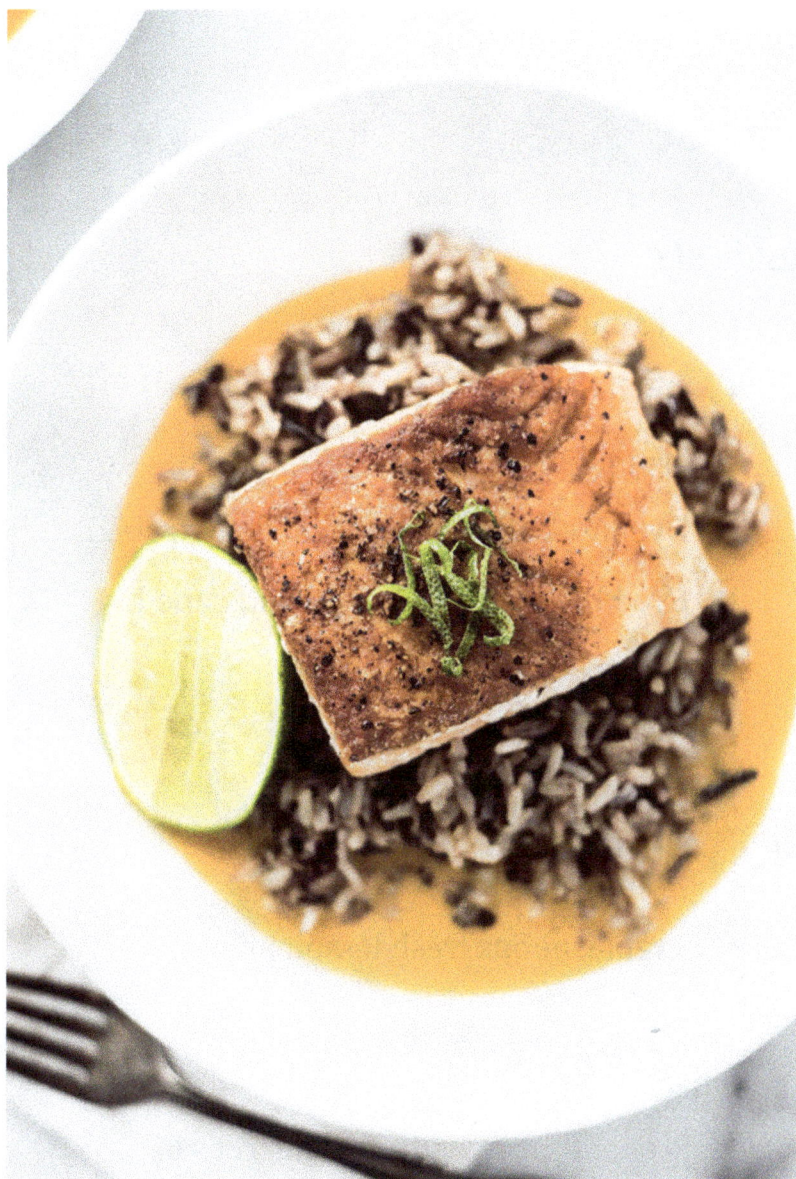

Salmon with Bell Peppers

Preparation Time: 15 minutes

Cooking Time: 20 minutes

Servings: 6

Ingredients:

- 6 (3-ounce) salmon fillets
- Pinch of salt
- Ground black pepper, as required
- 1 yellow bell pepper, seeded and cubed
- 1 red bell pepper, seeded and cubed
- 4 plum tomatoes, cubed
- 1 small onion, sliced thinly
- 1/2 cup fresh parsley, chopped
- ¼ cup olive oil
- 2 tablespoons fresh lemon juice

Directions:

1. Preheat the oven to 400 degrees F.

2. Season each salmon fillet with salt and black pepper lightly.

3. In a bowl, mix together the bell peppers, tomato and onion.

4. Arrange 6 foil pieces onto a smooth surface.

5. Place 1 salmon fillet over each foil paper and sprinkle with salt and black pepper.

6. Place veggie mixture over each fillet evenly and top with parsley and capers evenly.

7. Drizzle with oil and lemon juice.

8. Fold each foil around salmon mixture to seal it.

9. Arrange the foil packets onto a large baking sheet in a single layer.

10. Bake for about 20 minutes

11. Serve hot

Nutrition: Calories 220; Total Fat 14 g; Saturated Fat 2 g; Cholesterol 38 mg; Total Carbs 7.7 g; Sugar 4.8 g; Fiber 2 g; Sodium 74 mg; Potassium 647 mg; Protein 17.9 g

Shrimp Salad

Preparation Time: 20 minutes

Cooking Time: 4 minutes

Servings: 6

Ingredients:

For Salad:

- 1 pound shrimp, peeled and deveined
- Salt and ground black pepper, as required
- 1 teaspoon olive oil
- 11/2 cups carrots, peeled and julienned
- 11/2 cups red cabbage, shredded
- 11/2 cup cucumber, julienned
- 5 cups fresh baby arugula
- ¼ cup fresh basil, chopped
- ¼ cup fresh cilantro, chopped
- 4 cups lettuce, torn
- ¼ cup almonds, chopped

For Dressing:

- 2 tablespoons natural almond butter

- 1 garlic clove, crushed
- 1 tablespoon fresh cilantro, chopped
- 1 tablespoon fresh lime juice
- 1 tablespoon unsweetened applesauce
- 2 teaspoons balsamic vinegar
- 1/2 teaspoon cayenne pepper
- Salt, as required
- 1 tablespoon water
- 1/3 cup olive oil

Directions:

1. Slowly, add the oil, beating continuously until smooth.
2. For salad: in a bowl, add shrimp, salt, black pepper and oil and toss to coat well.
3. Heat a skillet over medium-high heat and cook the shrimp for about 2 minutes per side.
4. Remove from the heat and set aside to cool.
5. In a large bowl, add the shrimp, vegetables and mix well.
6. For dressing: in a bowl, add all **Ingredients** except oil and beat until well combined.

7. Place the dressing over shrimp mixture and gently, toss to coat well.

8. Serve immediately.

Nutrition: Calories 274; Total Fat 17.7 g; Saturated Fat 2.4 g; Cholesterol 159 mg; Total Carbs 10 g; Sugar 3.8 g; Fiber 2.9 g; Sodium 242 mg; Potassium 481 mg; Protein 20.5 g

Shrimp & Veggies Curry

Preparation Time: 20 minutes

Cooking Time: 20 minutes

Servings: 6

Ingredients:

- 2 teaspoons olive oil
- 11/2 medium white onions, sliced
- 2 medium green bell peppers, seeded and sliced
- 3 medium carrots, peeled and sliced thinly
- 3 garlic cloves, chopped finely
- 1 tablespoon fresh ginger, chopped finely
- 21/2 teaspoons curry powder
- 11/2 pounds shrimp, peeled and deveined
- 1 cup filtered water
- 2 tablespoons fresh lime juice
- Salt and ground black pepper, as required
- 2 tablespoons fresh cilantro, chopped

Directions:

1. In a large skillet, heat oil over medium-high heat and sauté the onion for about 4-5 minutes.

2. Add the bell peppers and carrot and sauté for about 3-4 minutes.

3. Add the garlic, ginger and curry powder and sauté for about 1 minute.

4. Add the shrimp and sauté for about 1 minute.

5. Stir in the water and cook for about 4-6 minutes, stirring occasionally.

6. Stir in lime juice and remove from heat.

7. Serve hot with the garnishing of cilantro.

Nutrition: Calories 193; Total Fat 3.8 g; Saturated Fat 0.9 g; Cholesterol 239 mg; Total Carbs 12 g; Sugar 4.7 g; Fiber 2.3 g; Sodium 328 mg; Potassium 437 mg; Protein 27.1 g

Shrimp with Zucchini

Preparation Time: 20 minutes

Cooking Time: 8 minutes

Servings: 4

Ingredients:

- 3 tablespoons olive oil
- 1-pound medium shrimp, peeled and deveined
- 1 shallot, minced
- 4 garlic cloves, minced
- ¼ teaspoon red pepper flakes, crushed
- Salt and ground black pepper, as required
- ¼ cup low-sodium chicken broth
- 2 tablespoons fresh lemon juice
- 1 teaspoon fresh lemon zest, grated finely
- 1/2-pound zucchini, spiralized with Blade C

Directions:

1. In a large skillet, heat the oil and butter over medium-high heat and cook the shrimp, shallot,

garlic, red pepper flakes, salt and black pepper for about 2 minutes, stirring occasionally.

2. Stir in the broth, lemon juice and lemon zest and bring to a gentle boil.

3. Stir in zucchini noodles and cook for about 1-2 minutes.

4. Serve hot.

Nutrition: Calories 245; Total Fat 12.6 g; Saturated Fat 2.2 g; Cholesterol 239 mg; Total Carbs 5.8 g; Sugar 1.2 g; Fiber 08 g; Sodium 289 mg; Potassium 381 mg; Protein 27 g

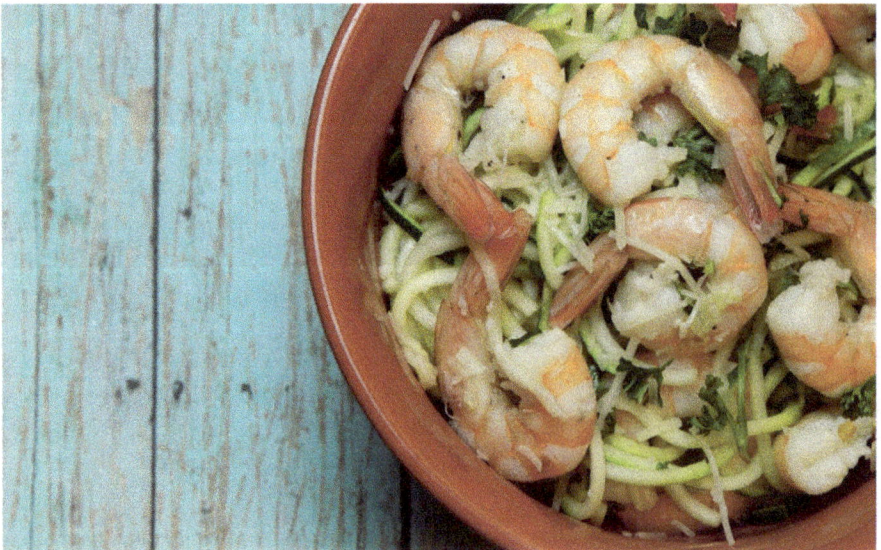

Shrimp with Broccoli

Preparation Time: 15 minutes

Cooking Time: 12 minutes

Servings: 6

Ingredients:

- 2 tablespoons olive oil, divided
- 4 cups broccoli, chopped
- 2-3 tablespoons filtered water
- 11/2 pounds large shrimp, peeled and deveined
- 2 garlic cloves, minced
- 1 (1-inch) piece fresh ginger, minced
- Salt and ground black pepper, as required

Directions:

1. In a large skillet, heat 1 tablespoon of oil over medium-high heat and cook the broccoli for about 1-2 minutes stirring continuously.

2. Stir in the water and cook, covered for about 3-4 minutes, stirring occasionally.

3. With a spoon, push the broccoli to side of the pan.

4. Add the remaining oil and let it heat.

5. Add the shrimp and cook for about 1-2 minutes, tossing occasionally.

6. Add the remaining **Ingredients** and sauté for about 2-3 minutes.

7. Serve hot.

Nutrition: Calories 197; Total Fat 6.8 g; Saturated Fat 1.3 g; Cholesterol 239 mg; Total Carbs 6.1 g; Sugar 1.1 g; Fiber 1.6 g; Sodium 324 mg; Potassium 389 mg; Protein 27.6 g

Pork Chop Diane

Preparation Time: 10 minutes

Cooking Time: 20 minutes

Serving: _4_

Ingredients:

- ¼ cup low-sodium chicken broth
- 1 tablespoon freshly squeezed lemon juice
- 2 teaspoons Worcestershire sauce
- 2 teaspoons Dijon mustard
- 4 (5-ounce) boneless pork top loin chops
- 1 teaspoon extra-virgin olive oil
- 1 teaspoon lemon zest
- 1 teaspoon butter
- 2 teaspoons chopped fresh chives

Directions:

1. Blend together the chicken broth, lemon juice, Worcestershire sauce, and Dijon mustard and set it aside.
2. Season the pork chops lightly.

3. Situate large skillet over medium-high heat and add the olive oil.

4. Cook the pork chops, turning once, until they are no longer pink, about 8 minutes per side.

5. Put aside the chops.

6. Pour the broth mixture into the skillet and cook until warmed through and thickened, about 2 minutes.

7. Blend lemon zest, butter, and chives.

8. Garnish with a generous spoonful of sauce.

Nutrition: 200 Calories; 8g Fat; 1g Carbohydrates

Autumn Pork Chops with Red Cabbage and Apples

Preparation Time: 15 minutes

Cooking Time: 30 minutes

Serving*: 4*

Ingredients:

- ¼ cup apple cider vinegar
- 2 tablespoons granulated sweetener
- 4 (4-ounce) pork chops, about 1 inch thick
- 1 tablespoon extra-virgin olive oil
- ½ red cabbage, finely shredded
- 1 sweet onion, thinly sliced
- 1 apple, peeled, cored, and sliced
- 1 teaspoon chopped fresh thyme

Directions:

1. Scourge together the vinegar and sweetener. Set it aside.

2. Season the pork with salt and pepper.

3. Position huge skillet over medium-high heat and add the olive oil.

4. Cook the pork chops until no longer pink, turning once, about 8 minutes per side.

5. Put chops aside.

6. Add the cabbage and onion to the skillet and sauté until the vegetables have softened, about 5 minutes.

7. Add the vinegar mixture and the apple slices to the skillet and bring the mixture to a boil.

8. Adjust heat to low and simmer, covered, for 5 additional minutes.

9. Return the pork chops to the skillet, along with any accumulated juices and thyme, cover, and cook for 5 more minutes.

Nutrition: 223 Calories; 12g Carbohydrates; 3g Fiber

Chipotle Chili Pork Chops

Preparation Time: 4 hours

Cooking Time: 20 minutes

Serving: *4*

Ingredients:

- Juice and zest of 1 lime
- 1 tablespoon extra-virgin olive oil
- 1 tablespoon chipotle chili powder
- 2 teaspoons minced garlic
- 1 teaspoon ground cinnamon
- Pinch sea salt
- 4 (5-ounce) pork chops

Directions:

1. Combine the lime juice and zest, oil, chipotle chili powder, garlic, cinnamon, and salt in a resealable plastic bag. Add the pork chops. Remove as much air as possible and seal the bag.

2. Marinate the chops in the refrigerator for at least 4 hours, and up to 24 hours, turning them several times.

3. Ready the oven to 400°F and set a rack on a baking sheet. Let the chops rest at room temperature for 15 minutes, then arrange them on the rack and discard the remaining marinade.

4. Roast the chops until cooked through, turning once, about 10 minutes per side.

5. Serve with lime wedges.

Nutrition: 204 Calories; 1g Carbohydrates; 1g Sugar

Orange-Marinated Pork Tenderloin

Preparation Time: 2 hours

Cooking Time: 30 minutes

Serving: *4*

Ingredients:

- ¼ cup freshly squeezed orange juice
- 2 teaspoons orange zest
- 2 teaspoons minced garlic
- 1 teaspoon low-sodium soy sauce
- 1 teaspoon grated fresh ginger
- 1 teaspoon honey
- 1½ pounds pork tenderloin roast
- 1 tablespoon extra-virgin olive oil

Directions:

1. Blend together the orange juice, zest, garlic, soy sauce, ginger, and honey.

2. Pour the marinade into a resealable plastic bag and add the pork tenderloin.

3. Remove as much air as possible and seal the bag. Marinate the pork in the refrigerator, turning the bag a few times, for 2 hours.

4. Preheat the oven to 400°F.

5. Pull out tenderloin from the marinade and discard the marinade.

6. Position big ovenproof skillet over medium-high heat and add the oil.

7. Sear the pork tenderloin on all sides, about 5 minutes in total.

8. Position skillet to the oven and roast for 25 minutes.

9. Put aside for 10 minutes before serving.

Nutrition: 228 Calories; 4g Carbohydrates; 3g Sugar

Homestyle Herb Meatballs

Preparation Time: 10 minutes

Cooking Time: 15 minutes

Serving: *4*

Ingredients:

- ½ pound lean ground pork
- ½ pound lean ground beef
- 1 sweet onion, finely chopped
- ¼ cup bread crumbs
- 2 tablespoons chopped fresh basil
- 2 teaspoons minced garlic
- 1 egg

Directions:

1. Preheat the oven to 350°F.
2. Ready baking tray with parchment paper and set it aside.
3. In a large bowl, mix together the pork, beef, onion, bread crumbs, basil, garlic, egg, salt, and pepper until very well mixed.

4. Roll the meat mixture into 2-inch meatballs.

5. Transfer the meatballs to the baking sheet and bake until they are browned and cooked through, about 15 minutes.

6. Serve the meatballs with your favorite marinara sauce and some steamed green beans.

Nutrition: 332 Calories; 13g Carbohydrates; 3g Sugar

Lime-Parsley Lamb Cutlets

Preparation Time: 4 hours

Cooking Time: 10 minutes

Serving: 4

Ingredients:

- ¼ cup extra-virgin olive oil
- ¼ cup freshly squeezed lime juice
- 2 tablespoons lime zest
- 2 tablespoons chopped fresh parsley
- 12 lamb cutlets (about 1½ pounds total)

Directions:

1. Scourge the oil, lime juice, zest, parsley, salt, and pepper.
2. Pour marinade to a resealable plastic bag.
3. Add the cutlets to the bag and remove as much air as possible before sealing.
4. Marinate the lamb in the refrigerator for about 4 hours, turning the bag several times.
5. Preheat the oven to broil.

6. Remove the chops from the bag and arrange them on an aluminum foil–lined baking sheet. Discard the marinade.

7. Broil the chops for 4 minutes per side for medium doneness.

8. Let the chops rest for 5 minutes before serving.

Nutrition: 413 Calories; 1g Carbohydrates; 31g Protein

Mediterranean Steak Sandwiches

Preparation Time: 1 hour

Cooking Time: 10 minutes

Serving: *4*

Ingredients:

- 2 tablespoons extra-virgin olive oil
- 2 tablespoons balsamic vinegar
- 2 teaspoons garlic
- 2 teaspoons lemon juice
- 2 teaspoons fresh oregano
- 1 teaspoon fresh parsley
- 1-pound flank steak
- 4 whole-wheat pitas
- 2 cups shredded lettuce
- 1 red onion, thinly sliced
- 1 tomato, chopped
- 1 ounce low-sodium feta cheese

Directions:

1. Scourge olive oil, balsamic vinegar, garlic, lemon juice, oregano, and parsley.

2. Add the steak to the bowl, turning to coat it completely.

3. Marinate the steak for 1 hour in the refrigerator, turning it over several times.

4. Preheat the broiler. Line a baking sheet with aluminum foil.

5. Put steak out of the bowl and discard the marinade.

6. Situate steak on the baking sheet and broil for 5 minutes per side for medium.

7. Set aside for 10 minutes before slicing.

8. Stuff the pitas with the sliced steak, lettuce, onion, tomato, and feta.

Nutrition: 344 Calories; 22g Carbohydrates; 3g Fiber

Roasted Beef with Peppercorn Sauce

Preparation Time: 10 minutes

Cooking Time: 90 minutes

Serving: *4*

Ingredients:

- 1½ pounds top rump beef roast
- 3 teaspoons extra-virgin olive oil
- 3 shallots, minced
- 2 teaspoons minced garlic
- 1 tablespoon green peppercorns
- 2 tablespoons dry sherry
- 2 tablespoons all-purpose flour
- 1 cup sodium-free beef broth

Directions:

1. Heat the oven to 300°F.
2. Season the roast with salt and pepper.
3. Position huge skillet over medium-high heat and add 2 teaspoons of olive oil.

4. Brown the beef on all sides, about 10 minutes in total, and transfer the roast to a baking dish.

5. Roast until desired doneness, about 1½ hours for medium. When the roast has been in the oven for 1 hour, start the sauce.

6. In a medium saucepan over medium-high heat, sauté the shallots in the remaining 1 teaspoon of olive oil until translucent, about 4 minutes.

7. Stir in the garlic and peppercorns, and cook for another minute. Whisk in the sherry to deglaze the pan.

8. Whisk in the flour to form a thick paste, cooking for 1 minute and stirring constantly.

9. Fill in the beef broth and whisk for 4 minutes. Season the sauce.

10. Serve the beef with a generous spoonful of sauce.

Nutrition: 330 Calories; 4g Carbohydrates; 36g Protein

Coffee-and-Herb-Marinated Steak

Preparation Time: 2 hours

Cooking Time: 10 minutes

Serving*: 3*

Ingredients:

- ¼ cup whole coffee beans
- 2 teaspoons garlic
- 2 teaspoons rosemary
- 2 teaspoons thyme
- 1 teaspoon black pepper
- 2 tablespoons apple cider vinegar
- 2 tablespoons extra-virgin olive oil
- 1-pound flank steak, trimmed of visible fat

Directions:

1. Place the coffee beans, garlic, rosemary, thyme, and black pepper in a coffee grinder or food processor and pulse until coarsely ground.

2. Transfer the coffee mixture to a resealable plastic bag and add the vinegar and oil. Shake to combine.

3. Add the flank steak and squeeze the excess air out of the bag. Seal it. Marinate the steak in the refrigerator for at least 2 hours, occasionally turning the bag over.

4. Preheat the broiler. Line a baking sheet with aluminum foil.

5. Pull the steak out and discard the marinade.

6. Position steak on the baking sheet and broil until it is done to your liking.

7. Put aside for 10 minutes before cutting it.

8. Serve with your favorite side dish.

Nutrition: 313 Calories; 20g Fat; 31g Protein

www.ingramcontent.com/pod-product-compliance
Lightning Source LLC
Chambersburg PA
CBHW050746030426
42336CB00012B/1688